YOU CAN STOP SMOKING NOW

(AND STAY STOPPED FOREVER)

YOU CAN STOP SMOKING NOW

(AND STAY STOPPED FOREVER)

ISBN1434841375
EAN-139781434841377

Third Edition 2011
First Edition 1995

IMPORTANT DISCLAIMERS

- This book and the processes therein are complementary to medical and psychological resources. As such they are not intended to serve as substitutes for proper medical or psychological care.
- The processes in this book cannot stop a person from smoking who honestly wishes to continue to smoke or chew tobacco – you must WANT to stop smoking.
- Smoking of any kind, including smoking marijuana, cocaine, or any other substance will negate the positive outcome expected from this book. To make this program work, you must stop smoking any and all substances. I hope this would be obvious.

YOU CAN STOP SMOKING NOW

Table of Contents

YOU CAN STOP SMOKING NOW

Why This Book?

In 1999, I moved my private practice into the offices of a physician. He and others often referred clients to me to stop smoking as it was a primary concern for most physicians and for those seeing their physician.

My physician colleagues wanted to refer their patients to someone sure to help their patients stop smoking. I wanted a process we could count on with any patient.

As a hypnotherapist trained in Neuro-Linguistics, Emotional Freedom Technique, and Rapid Eye Technology, I had many effective tools for assisting clients to make substantive life changes, including smoking cessation.

During my years of work at the Rapid Eye Institute, I became convinced that one must get to the cause of an addiction to effectively address it. And that seemed to bare out over my years of work with hundreds of clients there.

Since then, I learned that neurologically, an event held in memory is often represented repeatedly by subsequent similar events. Depleting the emotional energy from any event along the path of a "belief string" or neurological line of associated memories would effectively take me to cause. In other words, shaking one end of the line would effectively shake the other end as well.

YOU CAN STOP SMOKING NOW

For some time, I realized great success with clients simply by desensitizing recent events representative of their overall complaint. When it came to smoking, I would simply hypnotically regress the client to a more recent representative event, desensitize it of emotional energy, and then using hypnotic regression, extend that flattened energy to cause. Many clients responded positively to the technique.

I wanted a process that would do 3 additional important things:

1. Do away with withdrawal symptoms
2. Make cessation permanent
3. Work with 95+% of clients who came to see me.

From Fears Consulting to Smoking Cessation

In 2003, I made the professional decision to focus my practice in the area with the highest incidence of success – irrational fears. As a result, I dealt with hundreds of clients reporting irrational fears – fear of driving on the freeway, flying in jct aircraft, being in closed areas, elevators – the full range of fears. My success rate with irrational fears was very close to 100%. That is to say, almost 100% of clients coming to see me about an irrational fear lost their fear within a very short period of time – usually in one session. And their fears stayed gone.

That's a pretty good record.

YOU CAN STOP SMOKING NOW

A colleague called me one day and asked why I was no longer doing smoking cessation sessions since most smokers keep smoking because they are afraid of what will happen if they stop.

I had not considered this angle. It had been many years since I had smoked and I had forgotten this very important aspect of smoking.

Consequently, I invited a physician friend to again refer patients to me for smoking cessation. I worked with fifty of these referred patients using my Fear Neutralization Process. ALL of them stopped smoking and did not take up the habit again after 2 years.

IT WORKED!

I was thrilled. I finally had a process that met all my goals:

- Near 100% success rate – that is 100% of people coming to me to stop smoking would stop smoking in one or two sessions.
- The process would eliminate withdrawal symptoms completely or at least enough to adequately strengthen will-power so as to make abstinence easy.
- Near 100% of those who stopped would never take up the habit again – they would be non-smokers for life.
- I could teach my technique to my clients so they could be self-regulating. If they ever found

themselves wanting another cigarette, they could do a quick and easy process that would instantly eradicate the craving.

This book represents the process in book form that anyone can use.

Based on Emotional Freedom Technique (EFT), my Fear Neutralization Process stops cravings cold and is included in this book in the "Cravings Killers" section (the "20-Second Cravings Killer"). It's simple and easy to learn and do. It requires no products like CDs or cassette tapes. It requires no special skills and can be done by nearly anyone. No special equipment or knowledge is required.

The only requirement is a strong desire to stop smoking.

Just like eliminating irrational fears, my stop smoking program involves the physical body in a special way – addressing it as the valuable entity it is. Fear Neutralization respects the mind and the body together – building a successful partnership that helps one stop smoking and stay stopped forever.

You can do it.

I can help.

You Can Stop Smoking Now

Why Do You Smoke?

Your smoking habit may be understood as a natural function of the human brain. In effect, you have three separate brains within your skull that compete with each other for dominance. You have a left hemisphere, a right hemisphere, and a primitive animal brain called the midbrain or reptilian brain.

Generally, the purpose of the left hemisphere is to compute and figure - seeking answers to questions and fixing problems; the purpose of the right hemisphere is to plan, explore, and to question. The purpose of the animal brain is to survive - period. To that end, the animal brain seeks to enjoy pleasure and avoid pain. It is always evaluating every situation and environment in terms of benefit or threat (probabilities for pleasure or pain).

The animal brain generates survival signals that drive the body toward what it demands, such as oxygen, food, sex, and fluids. These survival needs are all associated with physical pleasure or pain - i.e., the better something feels, the more necessary it seems for survival and the worse something feels, the less necessary it seems for survival.

It doesn't matter how substances such as cigarettes get mixed in with the midbrain's real survival needs - the result is the same - a chemical dependency. Smoking is a chemical dependency.

YOU CAN STOP SMOKING NOW

Smokers self-medicate for a number of reasons – including social acceptance – but in the end, they are willing to jeopardize their health and the health of others to continue the use of that "medication."

Most smokers wish this was not so. They wish they could keep on smoking with impunity. But study after study has demonstrated without any doubt - continuing to smoke will severely weaken your body until you prematurely die - often with the terrible agony of lung, throat, or some other cancer. The "medication" is deadly - yet necessary for survival - at least that's what the animal brain part of you believes.

There is another brain that sits on top of the animal brain – the cerebral cortex. This "new brain," or neocortex, allows you to be conscious, to think, to have language, to control your voluntary muscles, and to solve abstract problems. Your neocortex is "you," and you are capable of defeating any appetite, even for oxygen or food. Anyone can stop breathing until unconscious or stop eating until dead.

Your voluntary muscles (hands, feet, etc.) are "wired" directly to your neocortex – to you. Your animal brain is unable to get what it wants without EXPRESS permission from YOU. It enlists your thoughts and intelligence, sees through your eyes, creates strong feelings, and persuades you to use your hands, arms, and legs in order to obtain its favorite substance – cigs. It must appeal to you to get nicotine into your bloodstream.

YOU CAN STOP SMOKING NOW

We use the neocortex, the human brain, our selves, to override the appetite for smoking. We call it "will power" and you have more than you may believe you have. You can control your habit without changing your religious beliefs, and without pursuing psychological improvements, moral or spiritual betterment, or labeling yourself in any way.

After all, you're a human being - with the POWER to control your animal urges!

Although your animal brain has no language ability, it uses your language and thinking centers to get what it wants. For example, if you wisely decide that smoking is bad for you, and that you will stop, you will soon hear that old, familiar voice telling you why you should continue smoking. You may even imagine a picture of yourself with a cigarette. That is your animal brain, expressing its demand for nicotine.

There are two parties to your addiction - you, and "it."

"It," the animal, is simply:

Any thinking, imagery, or feeling that supports smoking - ever.

"You," the reasoning, rational part, thinks:

The only reasonable and acceptable outcome of this program is to...

STOP SMOKING

FOREVER!!!

(You can do it. I can help.)

The Magic Bullet

First, let's investigate smoking cessation as a "program" - I'll bet you've quit smoking a few times and failed. That's why you want to try this program - in hopes it will be the "magic bullet" that will finally get you to quit.

So, let me tell you this up front -

IT'S IMPOSSIBLE TO
QUIT SMOKING!

Your animal brain is set up to WIN – and NOT LOSE. Quitting is Losing! Losing leads to dying and your animal brain is all about living – and not dying. To survive, you must continue – and NOT QUIT! That's why you can't quit smoking. Quitting smoking is tantamount to dying to your animal brain – and just like breathing, it will FORCE YOU TO CONTINUE – because quitting smoking is like quitting breathing.

So, let me say that again so you can really gestate on it:

IT'S IMPOSSIBLE TO
QUIT SMOKING!

But using your voluntary muscles, under the control of your neocortex...

YOU CAN STOP SMOKING!!
(and stay stopped forever!)

Why can't you quit but you can stop? Because stopping is a different command to the animal brain than quitting is. Quitting connotes dying. Stopping simply connotes stopping. You can stop walking without dying. You can stop blinking and not die. You can stop breathing (for awhile) and not die. Do you sense the difference yet? Your animal brain does!

And for this reason...

YOU WILL

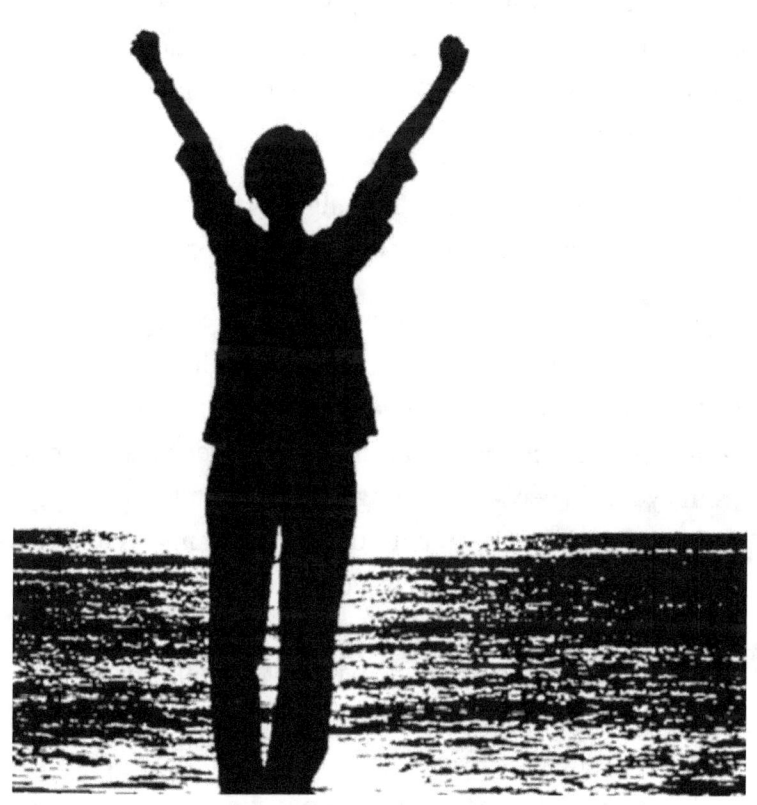

STOP SMOKING!!
(and stay stopped forever!)

You Can Stop Smoking Now

If It's So Easy, Why Can't You Stop?

You may ask, "Well, if it's THAT EASY, why don't I just tell myself to stop and be done with it?"

Because, my soon-to-be nonsmoker friend, "stopping" connotes "starting again" – so stopping is only the first step. I suppose you could simply stop over and over and over again until you completely release your need or desire for nicotine. But that's what you've already done – with the end result that you are still smoking.

I just want you to consider thinking in terms of stopping for now. We'll get to permanent change in a moment.

Right now, observe your thoughts and feelings, positive and negative, about smoking. ANY thoughts and feelings that support continued smoking are coming from "IT" – your animal brain; those that support abstinence are coming from you. When you recognize and understand your Animal Self, it becomes not-you, but "it," an animal – like a pet – that has been causing you to smoke. All "it" wants is pleasure. "I want a smoke," becomes, "It wants a smoke." Think to yourself, "I will never smoke again," and listen for its reaction. Your negative thoughts and feelings are your Animal Self talking back to you. Now, think, "I will smoke whenever I want." Your pleasant feelings are also the Animal Self, influencing your senses.

Your animal self communicates through sensations. It cannot speak, read, or write. It can only feel. And it communicates to you through sensation. Even emotions like anger, sadness, fear, and joy are all sensations so far as the animal self is concerned. Whenever you feel an emotion, you'll also feel some kind of sensation somewhere in your body – you may be so used to this that you don't consciously notice, but it is happening all the time.

For example, when you feel anger, you may clench your teeth or tighten your jaw (thus the word "tight-jawed" when referring to someone who is feeling angry). Generally speaking, your emotions are packages of sensations you've placed labels on. Then you put your marvelous evolutionary improvement – your neocortex – to work creating justifications to justify your sensations so you can have MORE OF THE SAME. "I'm angry because you called me stupid..." etc.

The animal self LOVES sensations. Sensations prove it is alive and ABLE to sense. Since survival is all important to the animal self, sensation becomes ultimately important to IT.

Actually, when you feel an emotion, you are feeling the results of chemical changes in your body that have created a set of sensations you labeled "anger" and to make the feelings okay – or justifiable – you assign those sensations to someone else's actions. By assigning a good reason to your feelings, you acknowledge and give your animal brain the okay to amplify the sensations – escalating your feelings.

In this example, your reasoning neocortex has been put to work giving your animal brain – IT – what IT wants. We do this ALL THE TIME and don't know we're doing it.

You Can Stop Smoking Now

The Magic of NOW, EVER, and NEVER

The magic words in stopping smoking forever are "Now," "Never," and "Ever," as in, "I will NEVER smoke again - EVER."

Now! The only time you can smoke is now, and the only time you can stop for good is right now. "I will never smoke again," becomes, "I never smoke now." It's not hard; anyone can do it – you can do it. Say it to yourself right now – "I NEVER smoke now."

Focus now on your own behavior and the consequences you experience from smoking.

Focus on the obvious.

If you're doing something harmful to yourself, wouldn't it be good to stop it? If smoking is killing you, wouldn't it be wise to stop?

Right NOW, experiment with the idea of never smoking again. NEVER!

How do you FEEL about NEVER – EVER – smoking again? – EVER!

What sensations come up for you?

What thoughts?

Consider your sensations – how intensely do you feel them? On a scale of 0-10 rate the intensity of EVERY sensation you feel RIGHT NOW as you consider NEVER EVER smoking again – EVER!

Now, with conviction – really mean it – say to yourself,

"I will NEVER – EVER – smoke again – EVER!"

Listen to your inner voices and sensations. What do they say?

To smoke or not to smoke. Ah, yes. That is the question! And listen to all the commotion in your head!

"If I could make this decision, I wouldn't have a problem in the first place. I could say never, but I would just be lying to myself. And if I say never, and then go ahead and smoke, I'll feel like a failure, so I would just be setting myself up for a big fall by saying never again. And even if I quit for good, how do I know my life would really be much better? I could see maybe six months, and if I was doing OK by then, it would be obvious that I would remain abstinent, because it would be stupid to start smoking again if things are going better because I'm not smoking. I might eventually have to give it up altogether, but right now I'm under incredible pressure from all sorts of things, and it wouldn't be good for me to undertake something as significant as a permanent commitment to stop smoking without really giving it some serious consideration and picking a time when things are going along more steady than they are right now. And actually, things can go on this way for a while, like I mean nothing really terrible is happening, and I can live with myself even if others can't. I know if certain things happen or if I get to feeling a certain way I will definitely smoke, so there's no use being perfectionist about this, and besides, I can cut back using techniques to control how much rather than whether I smoke. This abstinence stuff is probably good for people with problems that are more serious, or actually less serious than my problems. Maybe if I chew gum or use the patch, that will settle me down and make me cut back more reasonably than just stopping for good or maybe I should just get some support from my friends and maybe straighten some things out about me that are driving me to smoke. This commitment thing is too abrupt and there isn't really any proof it works, and the experts are really divided about the best way to approach smoking anyway. Actually the commitment to stop is probably the best idea of all, but it just doesn't come naturally, and there's no point in doing something unnatural because you can't live up to it down the line…"

"…blah, blah,"

SAID THE ANIMAL SELF!

Any sensations you feel – is the SAME VOICE!

YOU CAN STOP SMOKING NOW

....

*That voice and feeling is not you. It is
your voice talking to you from your*
Animal Self.

....

Your animal self is just doing its job. It intends to survive,
even if you do not.

Do you want to make a solid commitment? Are you ready
to take that permanent step into life?

You CAN do it NOW!

Let's review:

Your Animal Self is any thinking or feeling that supports
the possibility of any future smoking -- EVER.

You can't quit smoking. It's impossible.

You can stop smoking – and stay stopped forever.

There is only one possible time to make a commitment to
stop – and that time is RIGHT NOW.

The animal self, which resides in the midbrain, has no
perception of time. It lives as a timeless entity suspended in
eternity, with concept of time, and no memory except the
memory of pleasure and pain, and with no comprehension
of the future, functioning to survive in the endless now.

Therefore, now is never an acceptable time for the animal self to make a commitment to stop smoking. Just like now is never an acceptable time for the animal self to die - or experience pain or stop experiencing pleasure. Your animal self's only fear is of being deprived of what it takes to survive NOW. Its job, then, is to block you from depriving it of the cigarettes IT believes it needs RIGHT NOW.

So far, IT has been succeeding – you're still smoking.

If you wait until tomorrow, it will still be now to the animal self, only it will be then – and it will need a cigarette just as much as it does now.

The commitment to stop will be no easier to make then, than now – but it could be more difficult since the animal self is now aware of your desire to deprive it of what it wants.

The animal will do whatever it takes to convince you to return to giving it what it wants. It is totally amoral about it – not caring at all if it hurts someone in the process. It's not evil – in fact, it's totally non-judgmental about it.

IT is functionally immortal, and doesn't understand that you will die if you continue to smoke. To your animal brain, time is just a commodity to wear you down, to tire you out, to look for perfect opportunities, and to shorten the days, so that it will not suffer deprivation for long.

YOU CAN STOP SMOKING NOW

Are you ready to make a commitment to stop smoking forever?

It's entirely up to you.

But the only time you can do it is right now.

Why now?

Because it's always now, you know.

If you make a commitment to stop tomorrow, it will still be "now" then.

And once again, your animal mind will say, "Why now? Why never? Why can't we just think about this some more?" And you can keep coming back to the problem, forever – and in the meantime... you'll keep smoking... and killing yourself a little more each day.

Think it over.

You need not respond immediately.

But if you are ready...

Let's Do This NOW

This is not an experiment. We're not going to TRY this. We are going to DO this NOW! Trying is sure failure. Only DOING is going to DO.

A Commitment to Stop That WORKS!

Half-hearted plans to stop for good won't do. "Okay, I'll give it a shot." And "All right, I guess I'll give it a try." - won't DO! It's all or nothing, like jumping off the high dive. There's no turning back.

Now, think about the meaning of each of these six words, "I will never smoke again - ever."

"I" am in control of my muscles. Therefore, "I" call the shots.

"Will" is just my ability to make a decision, which requires no power.

"Never" means eternity, forever, to the last star in the universe.

"Smoke" is what I will never do.

"Again" which means that this decision is based on my past experience.

YOU CAN STOP SMOKING NOW

"Ever" reinforces and emphasizes the entire <u>commitment</u>.

Feel the discomfort. That is your animal brain, frightened of you, horrified at what you are planning.

Now, think about why you are stopping for good – focus on your reasons for stopping.

Feel the hope. Your reasons for stopping are not an illusion, a false hope, or a silver cloud. Those feelings are you in control of your animal brain. Trust those feelings of hope.

Now, say the words slowly to yourself, with as much meaning as you can, "I will never smoke again - ever." Mean it!

Consider your hands, which are necessary to pick up and hold a deadly cigarette.

Understand that your hands are under your complete conscious control at all times.

Your animal brain has no power over you; it is a quadriplegic that must appeal to you in order to convince you to smoke.

Wiggle your index finger.

Now challenge your animal brain to do the same. It CAN'T without your help. You have absolute control of your voluntary muscles. That's why they are called "voluntary"...

YOU CAN STOP SMOKING NOW

Ask yourself, "How bad (depressed, anxious, bored, angry, etc.) am I willing to get and still not smoke?"

(Here's a hint: Try, "As bad as I feel. That's how bad I can feel and still not smoke.")

Get it? It's a total commitment.

Listen for the echo!

When you state your commitment, you will almost certainly hear some serious commotion in your head.

It may be angry commotion, or sadness, or fear, or confusion, or bald cynicism like, "Oh, sure. A likely story. What a lie! What a load of crap this is!"

That is your animal brain in action, defending itself against the worst thing possible.

You are threatening it, in effect, with death.

Fortunately, IT is not you. And it won't die when you stop smoking.

You will survive, IT will survive. But for now, IT is certainly upset!

You must be willing to go the distance as necessary. And you CAN. And what will surprise you is how easy this commitment will be to keep. For now you must face IT with an absolute commitment.

YOU CAN STOP SMOKING NOW

Now, complete your commitment by saying again, with meaning,

"I will never smoke again - ever."

Only this time, add, "...and I will never change my mind - ever."

Your animal brain will get the message. Don't worry right now about the resistance and mind chatter you get. We'll take care of all that soon.

Congratulations on your commitment to stop smoking!

From here on, your task is simple.

All you do is recognize any thinking or feeling that even remotely suggests that you will smoke again.

Just recognize those feelings and thinking is the Animal Self, and they will fall silent. It's that simple!

Only when you engage in dialog with the Animal Self, will you get "white knuckles."

Stay alert for new animal activity, which may be sudden or gradual. It doesn't give up easily, and it is a strong opponent. When you feel it struggle within you, it is only your old friend having a hard time with its new master -- you. Your animal activity will taper off and within a matter of weeks or months abstinence will be totally effortless.

You Can Stop Smoking Now

With my process, however, your inner animal may have NO resistance at all to the new regime.

You will be surprised and fascinated at how much of your thinking is actually your Animal Self. You may be stunned to discover how much misinformation has become part of your Animal Self, paving the way for more smoking. In fact, your animal self will use whatever it takes to get you back under its influence. Just remember that you are the human in this relationship! IT is the animal, not you. And it is you who is in charge. This is important – YOU are in charge.

Allow yourself to naturally forget why you stopped smoking. Because you aren't going to smoke any more, no explanations are necessary to remain abstinent.

Let's Review

Using the language of the body - sensations - the body "speaks" to the mind - sometimes loudly - to get what it wants. When the rational mind says "no" the physical body simply increases its demands by increasing the intensity of the sensations until the rational mind gives in - usually causing the mind to create some kind of excuse or rationale for WHY it is doing something it KNOWS it doesn't want to be doing - like smoking.

To hedge its bets, the body will help the mind create irrational fears for what will happen if the mind chooses to stop the behavior - we call these "withdrawal symptoms" - which are VERY real - and the fear of experiencing those painful sensations keeps the mind in tow to the desires of the physical body. I call it "slave mentality" - and we all do it every day to some degree. It's why we have psychological defenses - they are our mind's way of rationalizing irrational behaviors that support the body's demands.

We are much more primitive than we like to consider ourselves. Most of the time, we are putting our big brains to work supporting the animal within us - the part that seeks pleasure and avoids pain - and explains why most people use little rational thought in what they do.

By making a solid and effective commitment to stopping smoking and stay stopped forever, you take charge of the body and set the stage for success. You may hear some grumbling and some resistance, but I'll show you a simple method to deal with them.

Between your commitment and dealing with the body's response to your commitment, you'll easily and effectively…

Stop Smoking

And

Stay Stopped Forever

YOU CAN STOP SMOKING NOW

How to Stop Smoking and Stay Stopped Forever

It may surprise you how easy it is to beat a smoking habit. MOST people who stop (estimates range around 75-80%) do so without any help from anyone or anything - they simply stop and that's that. Even "hardened" smokers can stop on their own - and often do.

That leaves me helping only about 20% of those who wish to stop.

My experience and belief is that 100% of those DETERMINED to stop will. It's not about whether or not you CAN – it's totally about whether or not you WILL.

That takes me to WHY. Why can't someone stop smoking when they want to? WILL, that's why. They don't have sufficient WILL to stop and stay stopped. My job is to help you strengthen your WILL to the point you can DO what you want when you want - stop smoking NOW – and stay stopped forever.

....

To remain a non-smoker, you must remain smoke free for AT LEAST 30 days.

....

Withdrawal symptoms for nicotine last only a couple days or so - never longer than a week. I will teach you how to diminish withdrawal to a nonentity so it is not an issue. But the HABITS associated with smoking can last much longer.

YOU CAN STOP SMOKING NOW

You must exercise adequate will power for some time after stopping to stay stopped.

There are basically two ways to strengthen the will to stop smoking:

One way is to approach the will mentally/emotionally. That is, with sufficient training and enough "buy in" by the person wishing to stop smoking. For example, the doctor tells the person they will die if they keep smoking because of the damage they will cause to their lungs and heart. This approach involves training by an authority (the doctor) and a buy in (the smoker gets scared enough to stop smoking).

There are problems with this method - it is prone to error and misinformation, and likely to fail in those with insufficient will already. They can always rationalize away important reasons to stop smoking - and then go on smoking even more convinced they CAN'T STOP - making stopping harder to do in the future.

The second way is to approach the smoking addiction physically - through the body. When the body (animal self) no longer NEEDS the substance of the habit, it will stop prodding the mind to supply its demand for it - cigarettes in this case. As long as the body BELIEVES it needs the substance for continued survival, IT will pressure the mind to continue supplying IT with the substance of its desire - tobacco in this case.

....

Remember - it is your rational mind that controls voluntary muscles like your arm and hand movements required to supply your lips with a cigarette...

When your rational mind says no with conviction, the arm and hand no longer move to the tune of the physical body - the animal within you must comply!

....

The body's need is determined by its <u>PAYOFF</u> - what does the body gain from the cig? I don't really care – it's your animal self's business. But we will use a special process to elicit those payoffs and then desensitize them until they no longer present a need. When the need is gone, so is the desire for the substance - and you are left free of the addiction.

The key to success with my approach to smoking cessation is in the way I elicit the physical body's payoffs.

We will desensitize those payoffs with a special desensitizing PROCESS. I've successfully trained hundreds of smoking cessation clients how to address their physical payoffs using a desensitizing process I'll teach you in this book. The process is NOT the key to success. Eliciting payoffs and making a commitment IS.

YOU CAN STOP SMOKING NOW

So, what is a physical body payoff?

Well, you know very well what it is - a sensation of pleasure. Since I can't determine for you what is or is not pleasurable for you (and incidentally, you can't either), I simply lump ALL SENSATIONS together as payoffs. As we discussed before, the body LIVES for SENSATION. When the body FEELS, it knows it's alive. And it is ALL ABOUT living - we call it survival - and it is priority numero uno to the body.

Addictions are all about pleasurable sensations - the body seeks pleasure and seeks to escape pain - which is why intensely pleasurable sensations are often accompanied by intensely painful consequences for stopping behaviors that bring about those pleasurable sensations. Fortunately, with my process, we will address both pleasurable and painful sensations together at one time leaving you neutral and without withdrawal symptoms.

Stop Smoking NOW!

The Plan

First, let's test your resolve by asking, "On a scale of 0-100%, how committed are you to stop smoking?"

Be honest with yourself. Anything less than 100% will undermine your commitment to stopping and staying stopped. You must be SURE you want to stop – because you WILL stop – and stay stopped.

You must stop smoking NOW and destroy any remaining cigarettes, cigars, pipes, and tobacco you might have at home, in the car, at work, wherever you've squirreled them away. I want you STRESSED out over this. Then we can get to work ending this problem and get you started on a path to full recovery.

When you are 100% sure you want to STOP for good...

Realize that you can NEVER EVER smoke another cigarette again - EVER!

Repeat this out loud to yourself with conviction,

....

"I can NEVER (emphasis!) EVER (emphasis!) have another cigarette - EVER! (double emphasis!!)"

....

Remember this commitment statement?

YOU CAN STOP SMOKING NOW

And now the MOST IMPORTANT PART –

While contemplating what it will be like to NEVER EVER have another cigarette EVER, what do you feel in your body?

Take an inventory of sensations - **list them ALL.**

If a thought pops up (like "Oh, my God, I can't live without my cigarettes") ask yourself, "...and when you're thinking that thought, where and how do you feel that in your body?"

Add your answer to the inventory list.

....

Remember – STAY PHYSICAL

....

Let's start by measuring your list

SUD – (**S**ubjective **U**nits of **D**istress) is a measurement scale from 0 (no distress) to 10 (maximum or unbearable distress).

Starting with the most intense feeling on your list, ask yourself, "On a scale of 0-10 with 10 being unbearable, how intensely do I feel [the sensation]?" For example, "How intensely do I feel the tenseness in my gut?"

Starting with the sensation with the highest SUD level, desensitize each sensation with my 20-Second Cravings

YOU CAN STOP SMOKING NOW

Killer found on page 37 or with Gage Work on page 40 or with the RET Quick Release process on page 42. Choose the process that works best for you.

Continue the sensation desensitizing process that works best for you until you can honestly report feeling completely free of sensations and intrusive thoughts when you state your commitment statement with full dedication.

Notes:

- *Feeling "good" or "well" or "satisfied" needs clarification in the physical - "How SPECIFICALLY do you feel 'good'?" - then process those sensations just as you would negative ones - in this case ALL SENSATIONS are considered part of the syndrome and MUST BE DESENSITIZED. When you are TOTALLY devoid of sensations around your commitment statement, you're done - but NOT BEFORE. This is critical to your success - don't let ANY physical sensation go unaddressed.*

- *Look for escape language - like, "maybe someday I can have one and be okay..." or "just one cig won't kill me..." or "I'll smoke my last one tonight..." or "it will still be okay for me to smoke a joint now and then..." or "I can still smoke a cigar/pipe and be okay..." - any other languaging that sounds like you will have another smoke. If you hear any of these, repeat the process on them - "And KNOWING you can NEVER, EVER have another cigarette EVER again, what sensations come up for you?"*

- *For most people, the 20-Second Cravings Killer (Fear Neutralization Process) works well to neutralize or desensitize physical sensations.*

YOU CAN STOP SMOKING NOW

Gather up ALL remaining cigarettes and destroy them right here right now. You may have to repeat your cravings killer process as necessary. It is YOUR life – so don't cheat!

Learn the cravings killer that works best for you by heart so you can desensitize your own physical sensations while you are not reading this. Having a tool you can use wherever and whenever a craving pops up will add a sense of self determination and help you build will-power.

2 important rules:

1. **Make sure you are 100% committed to stopping and staying stopped** - even if you are unsure you can do it yourself without help. You MUST BE committed to stopping and staying smoke-free.
2. **Attack the physical sensations** (body payoffs) rather than the mental/emotional parts. Sometimes that means investigating the mental attitudes and emotional elements as a means of identifying and addressing the physical sensations associated with them. **Always "get physical."**

Next, we'll look at the Cravings Killers you'll use to desensitize your fears, physical sensations, and intrusive thoughts about stopping smoking. These processes can be used to wipe out withdrawal symptoms altogether. They can also be used to eliminate the symptoms of other fears as well, including worries, frets, and irrational fears that keep you from enjoying your life fully.

I recommend that you use the Cravings Killers on every fear you feel, every intrusive thought that pops into your head, every craving, every hurt, every feeling you want to neutralize.

With the addition of one of the following desensitizing processes, you have a workable and effective plan for success. **ANY time you feel your animal brain piping up again, remember to simply do your process.** After a very short while, you'll no longer need to use the process.

Note: If in the future you feel the desire to return to smoking – perhaps due to unforeseen stresses, REMEMBER to do your process again. Don't wait to get home or to find a quiet place – DO IT RIGHT THEN AND THERE. If you simply cannot do your process (like you're in a business meeting or in front of a group, for example), then promise yourself you'll do it as soon as you can – then KEEP YOUR PROMISE!

Let's review:

1. State your commitment – and mean it!
2. Find those physical body sensations!
3. Desensitize them with a process!
4. Repeat as necessary.

Cravings Killers

(The key to staying stopped)

20-Second Cravings Killer

While focusing on your commitment to NEVER, EVER, smoke again – EVER...

Step 1 – Identify and describe in PHYSICAL terms[1] the most intense sensation you are feeling and where it is located in your body: "I feel tightness in my midsection." (Rather than "I need a cigarette." for example.)

Step 2 – Measure[2] the intensity of the physical sensation right now (0 = none, 10 = unbearable).

Step 3 – While rubbing the Sore Spot area with four fingers[3] speak out loud three times, "Even though I feel [physical sensation], I deeply and completely accept myself" For example, "Even though I feel this tightness in my midsection, I deeply and completely accept myself"

Step 4 - Using one or more fingers, rapidly and gently tap each of the points on the diagram 7-10 times each, starting from point 1 (eyebrow point) and ending with point 8 (collar bone point). While tapping each point, speak out loud, once at each point, a reminder phrase that assists you in keeping focus on the sensation. Example: "tightness"

Step 5 – After going through the tapping sequence of step 4, stop and measure the intensity of the sensation you are desensitizing.

- If the sensation drops to 0-1, return to your commitment statement and step 1 above to elicit more material to desensitize.

- If significant progress has been made, yet some sensation remains, while gently rubbing the Sore Spot area, return to step 3 and change the statement to: "Even though there is still some of this [sensation] remaining, I deeply and completely accept myself." Return to step 4 using the reminder: "remaining" - meaning "remaining [sensation]".

- If the intensity level is still not down to 0-1, ask yourself, "I still have this sensation because...?" Use the answer to that question to elicit deeper feelings. Remember – "stay physical". If you get, "because I feel anxious..." ask, "and when I feel anxious like this, how do I feel it in my body?" or "How does anxious feel in my body?" Then return to step 1 and repeat the whole process with this new sensation.

- If no progress has been made (SUD remains high), return to step 1 and explore what other sensations need to be addressed before this one will release. (Example: "I feel tight AND shaky in my midsection." Statement: "Even though I feel tight and shaky in my midsection I deeply and completely accept myself." Reminder: "tight and shaky"). Repeat steps 2-5.

Tapping Points: **Points**

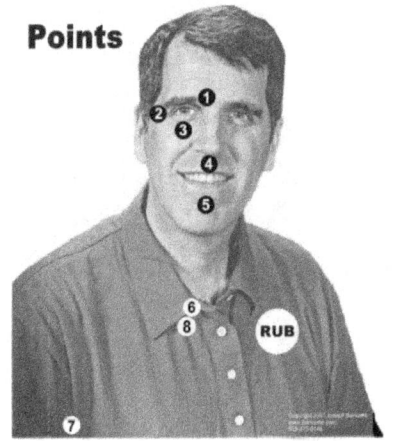

1. Inside edge of the eyebrow
2. On bone outside the eye
3. On bone under the eye
4. Under the nose
5. Between mouth and chin
6. About one inch down and out from top of sternum
7. Tender spot about 4 inches below armpit (bra line)
8. Same as point 6

Notes:
[1] Remember to STAY PHYSICAL. Use your own words as you would describe the sensations. Use words like "pressure" and "shaking" rather than "hurts" or "afraid".
[2] Known as SUD = Subjective Units of Disturbance or Distress (a 0 – 10 scale where 0=none and 10=unbearable)
[3] Sore Spot area - Place your hand over your heart. Where your fingers fall is the area. Often this area is tender to the touch.

[4] The order of tapping is insignificant. The order presented here is so you will more likely remember them all. You may tap on either or both sides if you wish. Tap hard enough to feel it but not so hard it hurts. Tap at a rate of about 3-4 taps per second.

Adapted from Gary Craig's Emotional Freedom Technique® (EFT). A video presentation of my version of the EFT process is available online at www.josephbennette.com/resources/therapies/eft.

Gage Work

10

This is an adaptation of a process developed by Astra Johnston, a therapist with the Lifeworks Group, Perth, Australia, GageWork may be thought of as using the metaphor of a "gage" or "meter" labeled with the name of a sensation. The gage itself is then "treated" with your favorite technique.

While focusing on your commitment to NEVER, EVER, smoke again – EVER...

Step 1 – Identify and describe in PHYSICAL terms the most intense sensation you are feeling and where it is located in your body: "I feel tightness in my midsection."

5

Step 2 – Measure the intensity of the physical sensation right now ——— 0 = none, 10 = unbearable.

Step 3 – Imagine a gage out in front of you that represents the intensity of your sensation. Give that gage a name – for example, "the nervous stomach gage." It can be vertical or horizontal.

Step 4 – Imagine removing the sensations from your body and place them onto the gage. Now the sensations belong to the gage. Just like a thermometer measures the temperature of the body.

0

Step 5 – Consider the gage. What would it take to make the gage go from its current level down to flat zero? For example, if you pulled out the plug in the bottom of a vertical gage, would the measurement fluid drain out and make it measure zero? Or, if a giant gorilla pulled your horizontal measurement needle from its current position down to the zero position, would that work? Imagine that SOMETHING pulls, drops, or otherwise makes the gage's indicator measure zero.

Step 6 – Once the gage has dropped to zero (and not before), imagine some device that will keep the gage at zero. Maybe placing a large boulder on top of the indicator needle will keep it at zero. Or maybe leaving the plug out of the bottom of the vertical gage will keep it from filling again. Whatever you choose, make sure it feels permanent to you.

Step 7 – Re-measure. Return to step 1 and test yourself again with your commitment statement. Repeat the process as many times as necessary to achieve a flat zero sensation level when you state your commitment with conviction.

Remember – focus your attention on the gage rather than your sensation. In effect, you will be transferring your sensation to the imagined gage. By dropping the energy of the gage, you'll automatically drop the energy of the sensation associated with it.

RET Quick Release

For more stressful material, or to do more than this simple process, go to www.rapideyetechnology.com or call 503-399-1181 to find a therapist in your area to work with.

1. While focusing on your commitment to NEVER, EVER, smoke again – EVER....
2. Identify and describe in PHYSICAL terms the most intense sensation you are feeling and where it is located in your body: "I feel tightness in my midsection."
3. Gage how much you feel it on a scale of 0-10 with 0 meaning not at all and 10 meaning unbearable.
4. Cast your eyes back and forth in a zigzag pattern while moving the zigzag up and down as long as you can before you either can't continue or you want to blink a lot.
5. Blink hard 3-4 times. Use your whole face.
6. Take three deep breaths, letting each out all at once in a sigh – emptying your lungs completely.
7. Gage again how you feel on the same 0-10 scale and notice the difference in the way you feel.
8. Repeat the process as necessary until the sensations are completely de-energized.

The RET Quick Release is copyrighted by Ranae Johnson, founder and owner of the Rapid Eye Institute, and is used here with permission.

Resources

Joseph Bennette, MRET, CHt
www.josephbennette.com

PowerStates
Promoting Empowered States of Mind
My blog
www.powerstates.com

1derWorks
www.1derworks.com
Feed Your Mind, Heal Your Body
Products for fun and growth

Oregon Hypnotherapy Association
www.hypnosis-oregon.com

The Rapid Eye Institute
Dr. Ranae Johnson, Founder
581 Lancaster Dr SE Suite 270
Salem, OR 97317-5642
503-399-1181
www.rapideyetechnology.com
(Please mention me when you call)

LifeWorks Group
Christine Sutherland, Founder
www.lifeworks-group.com.au
NLP Training, Research and Counseling, Consulting NLP

Starfields Network
Dr. Silvia Hartmann, Founder
www.starfields.org
EFT, EmoTrance, Project Sanctuary, Energy Hypnosis, Metaphysical
Fiction

About the Author

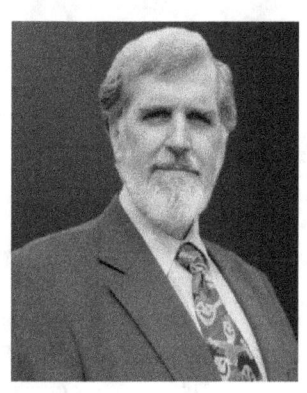

Joseph Bennette has trained thousands of people in Rapid Eye Technology, Emotional Freedom Technique, Hypnotherapy, and Life Skills. He has been a featured presenter at Northwest Hypnotherapy Conferences, Oregon Hypnotherapy Association meetings, on radio, television, and community events. Until retiring in 2007, Joseph had an active hypnotherapy practice in Salem, OR. He specialized in anxiety and anxiety-related emotions like panic, irrational fear, worry, fretting, and destructive self-doubt.

Joseph Bennette was trained in Rapid Eye Technology at the Rapid Eye Institute, Salem, OR, and holds a Master level certificate. He completed courses of study in hypnotherapy at the American Institute of Hypnotherapy, Santa Ana, California, and American Pacific University, Honolulu, Hawaii. He is also trained in Neuro-Linguistic Programming (NLP), Parts Therapy, Group Leadership, and Communication Technology. He is certified as a Clinical Hypnotherapist and is a member of the Oregon Hypnotherapy Association.

Joseph is the author of several books, numerous articles in trade publications, and is a frequent contributor to several online forums and email groups.

More
from Joseph Bennette

CDs:

- On the Threshold – Buy direct at
  https://www.createspace.com/1739901
- Emerging Evolution – Buy direct at
  https://www.createspace.com/1739917
- Inner Revisions – Buy direct at
  https://www.createspace.com/1739918
- NeuroGenesis – Buy direct at
  https://www.createspace.com/1716975

Books:

- Compassionate Healing, A Surrogate Approach – Buy direct
  at https://www.createspace.com/3338502
- Stop Smoking, And Stay Stopped Forever – Buy direct at
  https://www.createspace.com/3335721
- Read Faster, Quickly Improve Speed and Comprehension –
  Buy direct at https://www.createspace.com/3437983
- Oklahoma Story, Growing Up on Polecat Hill – Buy direct at
  https://www.createspace.com/3338639
- Carried Away, A Flight of Fantasy – Buy direct at
  https://www.createspace.com/3464432
- What Were You Thinking, Common Thinking Errors and
  What to Do About Them – Buy direct at
  https://www.createspace.com/3359869

Search Amazon.com for "Joseph Bennette"

You Can
Stop Smoking
NOW!
(and stay stopped forever)